The Perfect Cookbook for Autoimmune Disease Patient

25 Recipes Autoimmune Patients will enjoy

By

Heston Brown

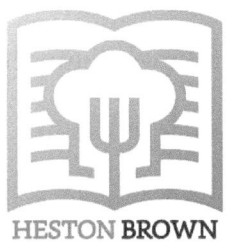

HESTON **BROWN**

Copyright 2019 Heston Brown

Thank you so much for buying my book! I want to give you a special gift!

Receive a special gift as a thank you for buying my book. Now you will be able to benefit from free and discounted book offers that are sent directly to your inbox every week.

To subscribe simply fill in the box below with your details and start reaping the rewards! A new deal will arrive every day and reminders will be sent so you never miss out. Fill in the box below to subscribe and get started!

https://heston-brown.getresponsepages.com

Subscribe
to our newsletter

Your Email

Table of Contents

Chapter I - Autoimmune Disease Beverage Recipes

xxxxxxxxxxxxxxxxxxxxxxxxxxxxxxxxxxxxxxxx

Recipe 1: Cucumber and Avocado Smoothie

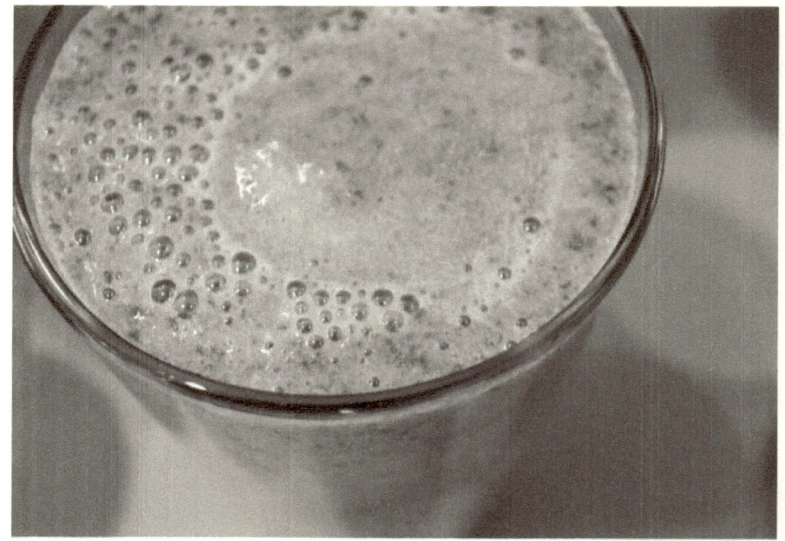

Why buy overpriced coffee that can aggravate autoimmune diseases when you can enjoy this delicious anti-inflammatory smoothie.

Yield: 1

Cooking Time: 5 minutes

List of Ingredients:

- 1 avocado, pitted and peeled
- 1 cucumber, peeled and sliced
- ½ cup coconut water
- 2 Tbsp. basil
- 2 Tbsp. lime juice
- 1/8 tsp. turmeric

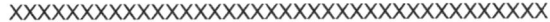

XXXXXXXXXXXXXXXXXXXXXXXXXXXXXXXXXXXXXX

Instructions:

Step 1: Place the avocado, cucumber, coconut water, lime juice, basil and turmeric in a food processor.

Step 2: Pulse the ingredients for several seconds until the mixture is smooth.

Step 3: If you want the smoothie to be chilled, add the ice cubes and pulse once again until the mixture is smooth. You can skip this step if you don't want the drink chilled or you chilled the ingredients before blending.

Step 4: Transfer the smoothie into a tall glass. Add a straw and enjoy immediately.

Recipe 2: Lemon Water

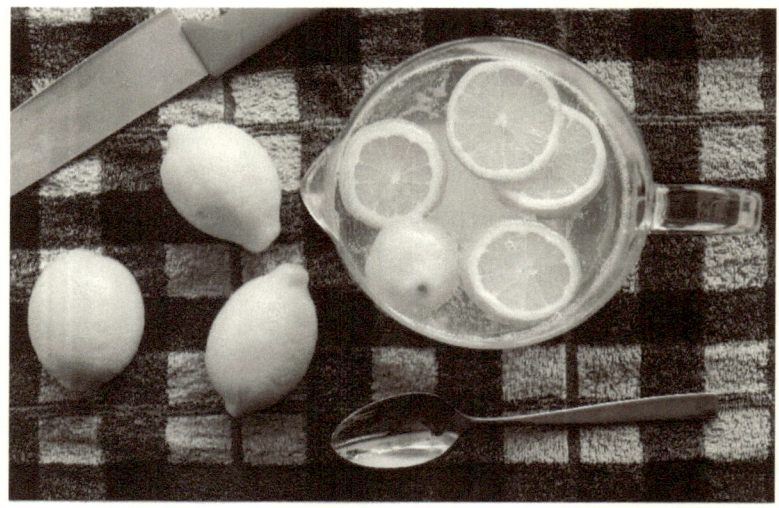

Some studies has shown that lemon water may have a positive effect on autoimmune disease. Furthermore, drinking lemon water is a tasty way to keep yourself hydrated and prevent inflammation.

Yield: 1

Cooking Time: 5 minutes + time to chill

List of Ingredients:

- ½ lemon
- 1/3 cup boiling water
- ¼ cup cold water

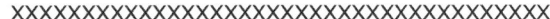

xxxxxxxxxxxxxxxxxxxxxxxxxxxxxxxxxxxxxxxx

Instructions:

Step 1: Hold the half of a lemon over a glass and squeeze until you cannot extract any more juice from the fruit.

Step 2: Carefully pour the boiling water into the glass and stir. Let sit for a minute or two.

Step 3: Pour the cold water into the glass and stir. Set the glass in the fridge to chill to the desired consistency. Drink the lemon juice with a straw.

Tips: You can alter this recipe by adding cucumbers or honey to taste. Furthermore, to prevent any damage caused by the acidicness of the lemon juice, rinse your mouth out with water after consuming the lemon water.

Recipe 3: Kiwi and Strawberry Smoothie

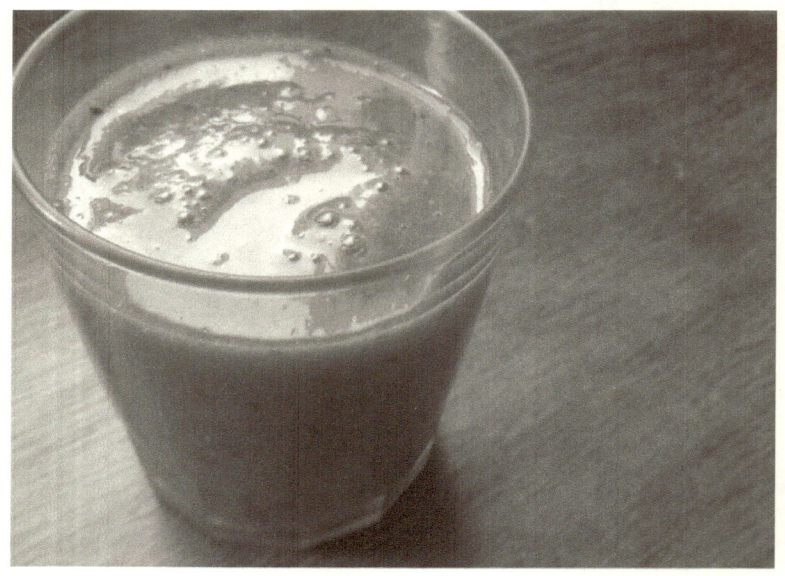

Delicious and fruity, this kiwi and strawberry smoothie works well as a quick, on-the-go breakfast drink or a snack.

Yield: 1

Cooking Time: 5 to 8 minutes

List of Ingredients:

- 1 cup strawberries, stems removed
- 1 kiwi, peeled
- 1 cup coconut water
- 2 cups baby spinach
- Juice from 1 lime
- 2 to 3 ice cubes, optional

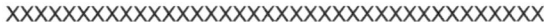

xxxxxxxxxxxxxxxxxxxxxxxxxxxxxxxxxxxxxxx

Instructions:

Step 1: Place all the ingredients into a blender or food processor.

Step 2: Pulse the ingredients for several seconds until the mixture is smooth.

Step 3: If you want the smoothie to be chilled, add the ice cubes and pulse once again until the mixture is smooth. You can skip this step if you don't want the drink chilled or you chilled the ingredients before blending.

Step 4: Transfer the smoothie into a tall glass. Add a straw and enjoy immediately.

Recipe 4: The Anti-Inflammatory Smoothie

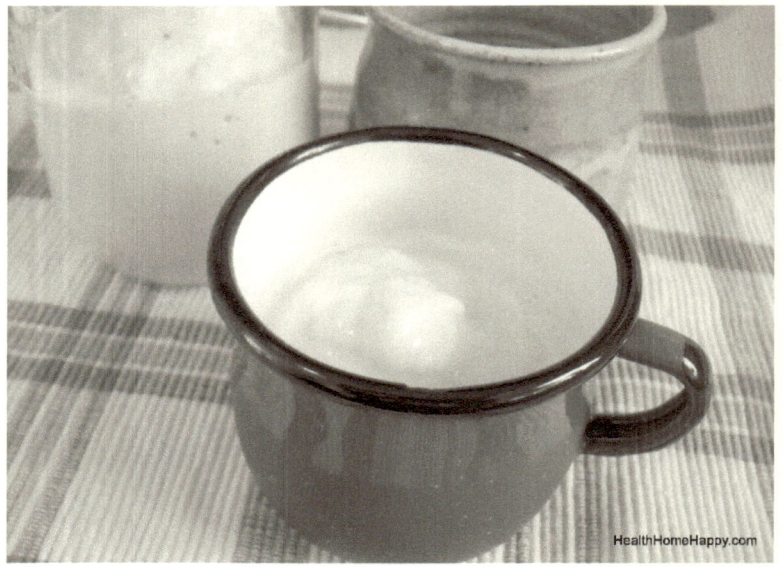

This delicious smoothie doesn't contain any of the common inflammatory inducing ingredients, such as flours, refined sugars and gluten, which are commonly found in overly processed foods.

Yield: 1

Cooking Time: 5 to 8 minutes

List of Ingredients:

- ½ ripe banana, peeled
- 1/3 cup spinach, frozen
- 1 cup raspberries, frozen
- Water

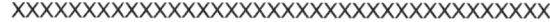

Instructions:

Step 1: Place the banana, raspberries and spinach in a blender or food processor.

Step 2: Pulse the ingredients for several seconds until the mixture is smooth. Add water to the mixture, a little bit at a time, until the smoothie reaches the desired consistency.

Step 3: Transfer the smoothie into a tall glass. Add a straw and enjoy immediately.

Recipe 5: Shake It Up

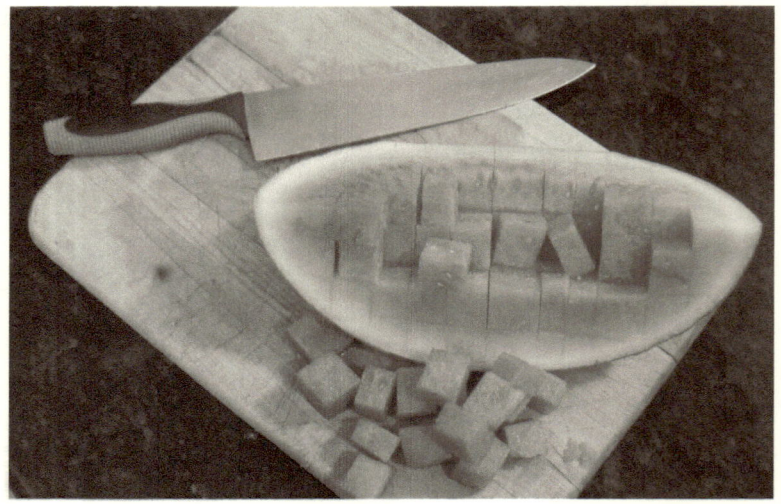

This watermelon shake will help satisfy even the most nagging sweet tooth without negatively effecting autoimmune diseases or inflammation.

Yield: 1

Cooking Time: 6 minutes

List of Ingredients:

- ½ cup coconut milk, unsweetened
- 1 cup watermelon cubes, seedless
- 1 Tbsp. coconut oil
- Juice from 1 lime
- 10 mint leaves
- 2 ice cubes

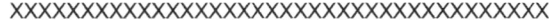

xxxxxxxxxxxxxxxxxxxxxxxxxxxxxxxxxxxxxx

Instructions:

Step 1: Combine the watermelon cubes, coconut milk, coconut oil, mint leaves and lime juice in a blender. Blend the ingredients until smooth.

Step 2: If you want the smoothie to be chilled, add the ice cubes and pulse once again until the mixture is smooth. You can skip this step if you chilled the ingredients before blending.

Step 4: Transfer the watermelon shake into a tall glass. Add a straw and enjoy immediately.

Chapter II - Autoimmune Disease Breakfast Recipes

xxxxxxxxxxxxxxxxxxxxxxxxxxxxxxxxxxxxxxxx

Recipe 6: No Oat Porridge

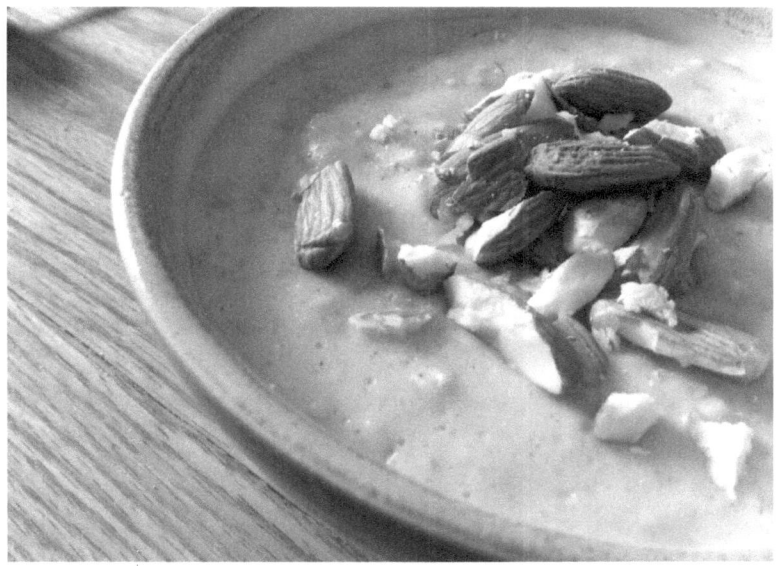

This porridge recipe ditches the oats and replaces it with cauliflower rice for an anti-inflammation breakfast meal.

Yield: 4 to 6

Cooking Time: 20 to 30 minutes

List of Ingredients:

- 40 grams unsweetened shredded coconut
- 40 grams cauliflower rice
- 200 grams apple, grated
- ½ tsp. ground cinnamon
- Tin of coconut milk
- 1 tsp. vanilla
- Raw honey, to taste

xxxxxxxxxxxxxxxxxxxxxxxxxxxxxxxxxxxxxxx

Instructions:

Step 1: Stir the coconut, cauliflower rice, grated apple, cinnamon, coconut milk and vanilla together in a pan until well mixed.

Step 2: Set the pan on the stove over high heat and then bring the mixture to a boil. Once it begins to boil, reduce the heat and allow the porridge to simmer for about 20 minutes.

Step 3: Remove the pan from heat and let cool. Stir in the raw honey to taste before serving.

Tip: Porridge can be served hot or cold.

Recipe 7: Breakfast Sausage

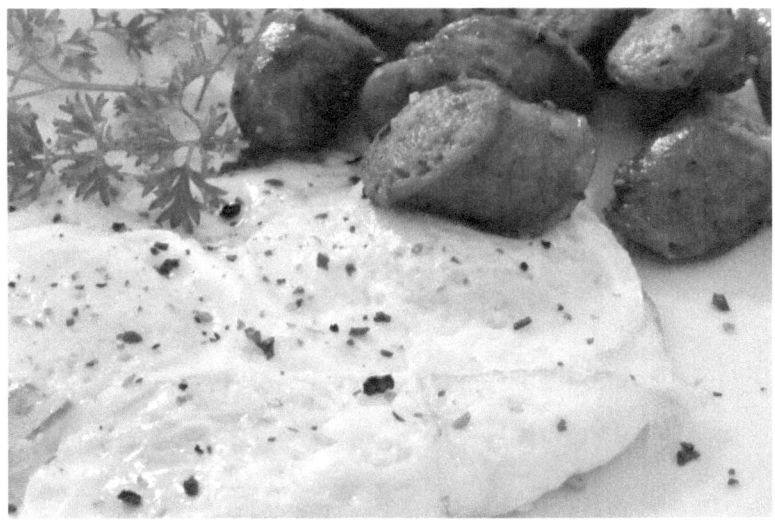

This delicious breakfast sausage features apples and chicken for a unique and health meal.

Yield: 12 patties

Cooking Time: 40 to 45 minutes

List of Ingredients:

- 1-pound ground chicken
- 1 apple, peeled, cored and diced finely
- 3 Tbsp. parsley, diced
- 1 Tbsp. thyme leaves, diced
- 1 Tbsp. oregano, diced
- 2 tsp. garlic power
- Sea salt, to taste
- Ground black pepper, to taste
- Coconut oil

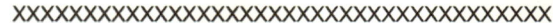

xxxxxxxxxxxxxxxxxxxxxxxxxxxxxxxxxxxxxxxxx

Instructions:

Step 1: Turn the oven to 425-degrees and let preheat. Line the bottom of a baking tray with foil.

Step 2: Add some coconut oil to a medium-sized skillet. Set the skillet on the stove over medium heat and let the oil warm up a bit.

Step 3: Stir together the thyme, apples, oregano and parsley before transferring them into the skillet. Sauté the mixture for about 8 minutes.

Step 4: Remove the skillet from heat and let cool for a few minutes. Dump the mixture into a bowl.

Step 5: Add the ground chicken to the bowl and knead with your hands until well mixed. Season the mixture with salt, pepper and garlic powder and knead once again for a few more minutes.

Step 6: Using your hands, form 12 patties from the chicken mixture in Step 5. Lay the patties on the prepared tray from Step 1.

Step 7: Bake the patties in the preheated oven for about 25 minutes, flipping the patties over halfway through the baking process.

Step 8: Let the patties cool a bit before serving.

Chapter III - Autoimmune Disease Lunch Recipes

xxxxxxxxxxxxxxxxxxxxxxxxxxxxxxxxxxxxxxxx

Recipe 8: Fake Sushi

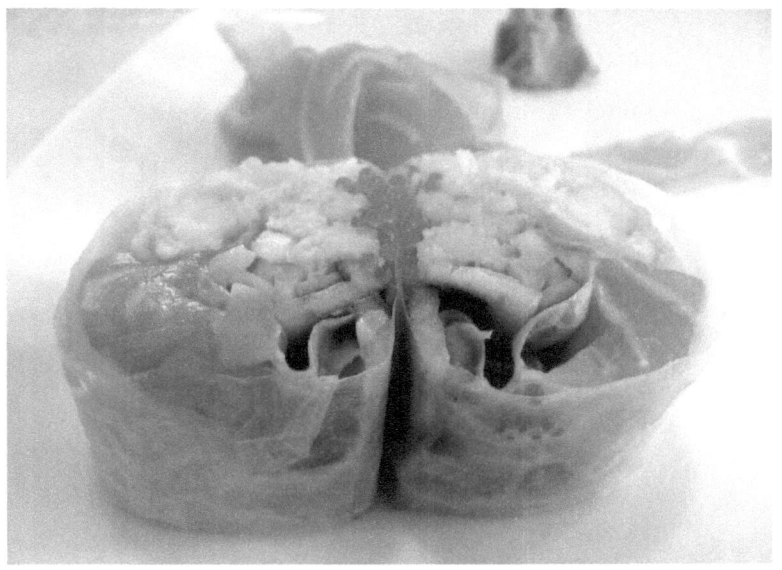

This fake sushi uses cucumbers to provide you with a refreshing and tasty lunch that won't aggravate inflammation and autoimmune diseases.

Yield: 2

Cooking Time: 50 to 60 minutes

List of Ingredients:

- 1 cucumber, peeled
- 1 carrot, peeled
- 8 ounces salmon
- 4 sheets of nori (seaweed sheets for sushi)
- 2 avocadoes, mashed
- ½ cup watercress

xxxxxxxxxxxxxxxxxxxxxxxxxxxxxxxxxxxxxxxxxx

Instructions:

Step 1: Prepare the cucumber and carrot by cutting it carefully into thin strips. Do the same with the salmon.

Step 2: Lay the 4 nori sheets out flat on a level surface. Make sure the seaweed sheets are laying with the shiny side facing downward.

Step 3: Spread about a fourth of the avocado over the 4 nori sheets. Lay ¼ of the cucumber, carrot and salmon strips in the middle of each sheet.

Step 4: Using the avocado pasta as a sort of glue, tightly roll the seaweed sheets as you would if you were making traditional sushi.

Step 5: Place the fake sushi in the fridge for about 30 minutes. Slice the sushi into pieces before serving.

Recipe 9: Burrito Bowl

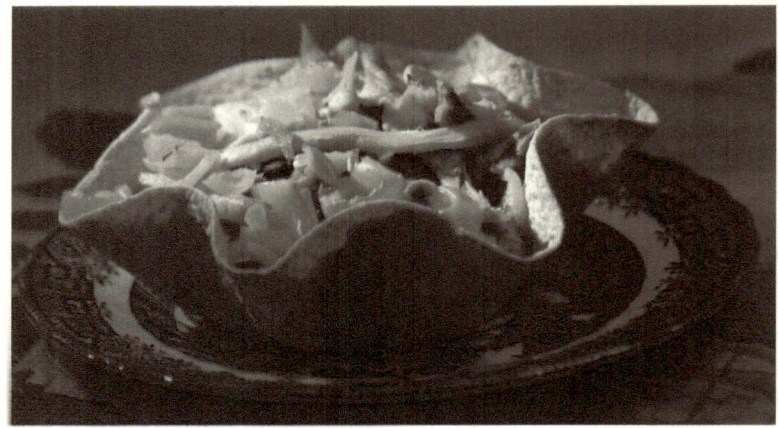

This vegan-take on the traditional burrito bowl is delicious, gluten-free and compliant with the autoimmune disease diet.

Yield: 2 to 4

Cooking Time: 40 to 45 minutes

Quinoa Ingredients:

- 1 cup quinoa
- ½ tsp. sea salt

Kale Ingredients:

- 1 bunch kale, destemmed and chopped finely
- 2 Tbsp. extra-virgin olive oil
- ½ cup lemon juice
- ½ tsp. cumin
- ½ jalapeno pepper, chopped finely
- Sea salt, to taste

Avocado Salsa Ingredients:

- 2 tomatoes, diced
- 1 avocado, sliced
- 1 jalapeno pepper, diced
- ¼ red onion, chopped finely
- ½ cup cilantro leaves, diced
- 1 lemon

Black Beans Ingredients:

- 2 cans black beans, rinsed and drained
- 2 garlic cloves, minced
- ½ red onion, diced finely
- ¼ tsp. chili powder

xxxxxxxxxxxxxxxxxxxxxxxxxxxxxxxxxxxxxxxxxx

Instructions:

Step 1: Make the quinoa by bring the water to a boil before stirring in the uncooked quinoa and the salt. Reduce the heat and let the mixture simmer for about 25 minutes. If needed, season the cooked quinoa with salt and pepper. Set the cooked quinoa to the side for the moment.

Step 2: Next, prepare the kale salad by mixing the olive oil, lemon juice, salt, cumin and jalapeno together. This is the dressing. Place the kale in a bowl and drizzle the dressing over top. Toss to evenly coat the kale with the dressing. Set to the side for the moment.

Step 3: In a small bowl, mix all the ingredients listed under the avocado salsa. Set to the side for the moment.

Step 4: Cook the beans by heating 1 Tbsp. of olive oil in a saucepan and set on the stove over medium heat. Add the garlic, onion and sauté for 5 minutes. Stir in the chili powder and the beans, and cook until the beans are tender.

Step 5: Divide the quinoa, kale salad and beans between serving bowls. Add some of the avocado salsa to the top and serve.

Recipe 10: Beef Teriyaki Stir fry

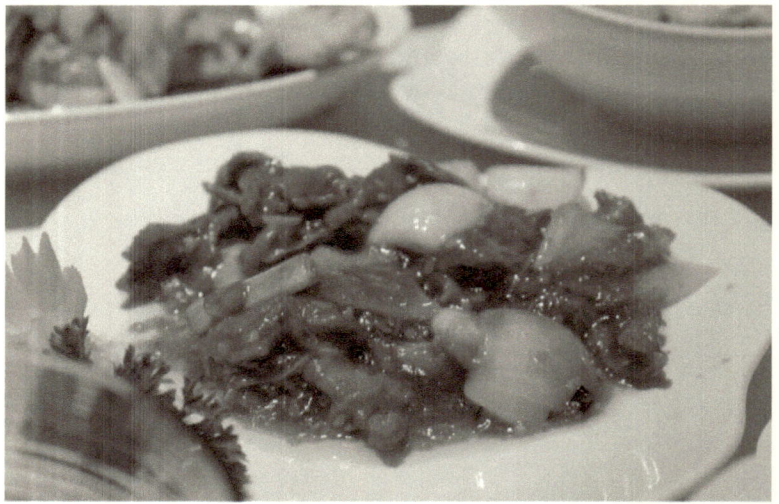

This autoimmune disease diet take on the traditional Oriental dish is so tasty that you would never guess that it was designed with a special diet in mind.

Yield: 2 to 3

Cooking Time: 35 to 45 minutes

List of Ingredients:

- 2 Tbsp. coconut oil
- ½ cup coconut aminos
- 2 garlic cloves, minced
- 3 Tbsp. raw honey
- 1 tsp. ginger, grated
- ½ tsp. fish sauce
- 1 Tbsp. Sriracha
- 2 Tbsp. arrowroot powder
- 1 tsp. sesame oil
- 1 seeded and thinly sliced green bell pepper
- 1 seeded and thinly sliced red bell pepper
- 1 cup mushrooms, thinly sliced
- 1-pound flank steak, fat trimmed and thinly sliced
- Salt, to taste
- Ground black pepper, to taste
- Chives, for garnish

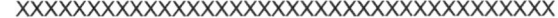

xxxxxxxxxxxxxxxxxxxxxxxxxxxxxxxxxxxxxxxx

Instructions:

Step 1: Set a skillet on the stove over medium heat and add the coconut oil. Let the skillet and the oil heat for several seconds.

Step 2: Place the ginger and the minced garlic cloves in the skillet and let sauté until tender. Turn the heat down to low.

Step 3: Add the coconut aminos and stir until well incorporated. Turn the heat up a bit before stirring in the sesame oil, fish sauce, honey and sriracha. Let the mixture start to boil.

Step 4: Carefully pour a little of the arrowroot powder into the mixture and whisk until well incorporated. Continue in this manner until you have whisked in all the arrowroot powder.

Step 5: Stir in the green pepper, red pepper, onion and mushrooms. Let the mixture simmer for about 10 minutes.

Step 6: Transfer the mixture into a mixing bowl before setting the skillet back on the stove.

Step 7: Turn the heat up to medium before laying the steak slices along the bottom of the skillet. Cook the steak for about 4 minutes on each side.

Step 8: Place the vegetable mixture from Step 6 into the skillet with the steak slices and stir until well combined.

Step 9: Remove the skillet from heat and garnish with the chives before dishing the stir fry out onto a serving plate.

Recipe 11: Lentil Cakes

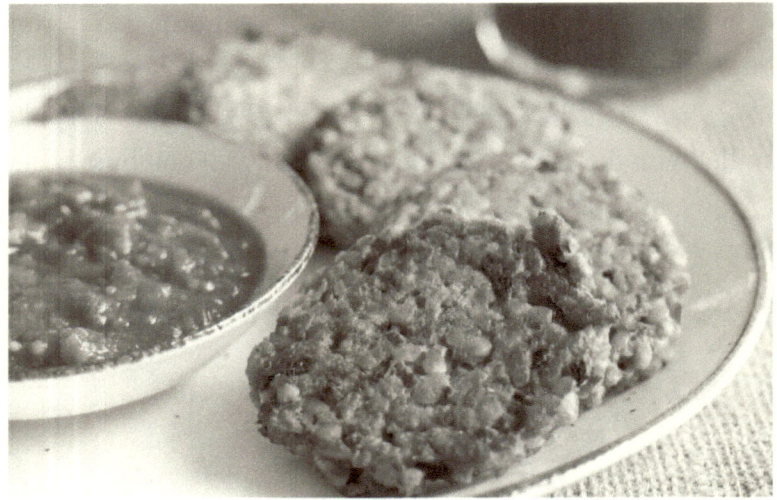

This delicious lunch recipe can be served alone or on top of salad.

Yield: 8

Cooking Time: 55 to 60 minutes

List of Ingredients:

- 1 cup lentils, dry
- 2 ½ cups water
- ½ cup walnuts, chopped
- 1 cup almonds or cashews, crushed
- ¼ cup coconut milk
- ½ yellow onion, minced
- 2 large eggs, slightly beaten
- 1 tsp. onion powder
- 2 Tbsp. coconut oil
- 1 cup ground flaxseed
- Salt, to taste
- Ground black pepper, to taste

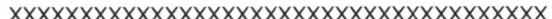

xxxxxxxxxxxxxxxxxxxxxxxxxxxxxxxxxxxxxxx

Instructions:

Step 1: Pour the water into a pot and set the pot on the stove over high heat. Add the lentils and let the water boil. Once boiling, turn the heat down to low, cover the pot and let the lentils cook for about 30 minutes. After the allotted time, drain the water from the cooked lentils before transferring them into a mixing bowl.

Step 2: Add the coconut milk, crushed nuts, eggs, onion and walnuts into the mixing bowl with the cooked lentils. Use your hands to knead the mixture for several minutes. Season with the onion powder and mix once again with your hands.

Step 3: Set the mixing bowl to the side and let the mixture rest for about 30 minutes.

Step 4: While the mixture is resting, place the coconut oil into a skillet and set the skillet on the stove over medium heat.

Step 5: Using your hands, shape the mixture into balls and roll in the ground flaxseed. Flatten the coated balls into a patty shape and fry one each side, about 6 minutes for each side.

Recipe 12: Garlic Saffron Cauliflower

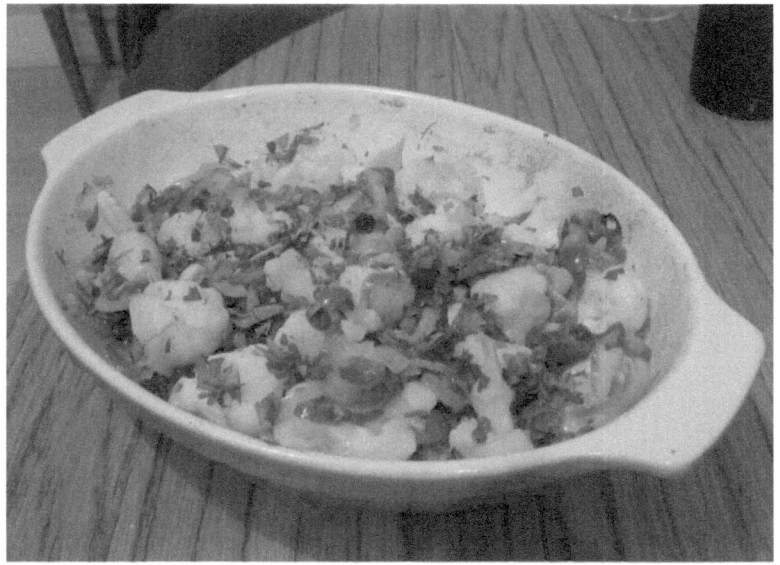

This cauliflower recipe is flavored with garlic and saffron and can be used as a single lunch meal or side dish.

Yield: 4

Cooking Time: 25 to 30 minutes

List of Ingredients:

- 1 cauliflower head, diced
- 2 cups vegetable stock, low sodium
- 2 Tbsp. extra-virgin olive oil
- 2 shallots, sliced thinly
- 5 garlic cloves, minced
- 1 tsp. salt
- Pinch saffron

xxxxxxxxxxxxxxxxxxxxxxxxxxxxxxxxxxxxxx

Instructions:

Step 1: Pour the vegetable stock into a pot and set on the stove over high heat. Let the stock boil before stirring in the chopped cauliflower and allowing it to boil for about 8 minutes.

Step 2: While the cauliflower is cooking, heat the olive oil in a skillet. Once the oil is hot, add the shallots, garlic and saffron and let sauté for about 6 minutes.

Step 3: Strain the vegetable stock from the cauliflower, making sure to reserve the liquid. Place the cooked cauliflower into a mixing bowl.

Step 4: Scoop out about half of the reserved liquid and add it to the cauliflower. Add the shallot mixture from Step 2.

Step 5: Mash the mixture with a potato masher until you achieve the desired texture.

Chapter IV - Autoimmune Disease Soup and Salad Recipes

xxxxxxxxxxxxxxxxxxxxxxxxxxxxxxxxxxxxxxxx

Recipe 13: Salmon and Strawberry Salad

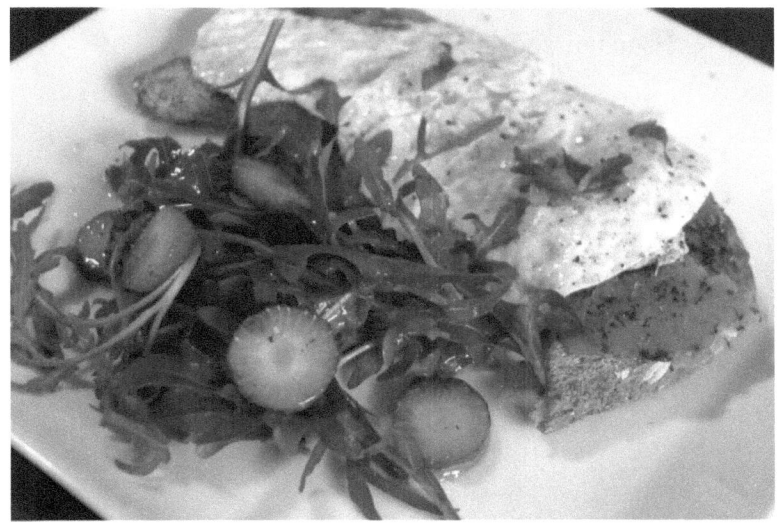

Forget traditional and boring salads with this delicious salmon and strawberry dish that won't aggravate autoimmune conditions or cause inflammation.

Yield: 2

Cooking Time: 20 to 25 minutes

List of Ingredients:

- 12 ounces salmon fillets, sliced in two
- 1 cup strawberries, de-stemmed and sliced
- 2 cups mixed salad greens
- 1 avocado, peeled and cubed
- 2 Tbsp. balsamic vinegar, unsweetened
- 2 Tbsp. olive oil, extra-virgin
- 1 Tbsp. lemon juice
- Salt, optional

xxxxxxxxxxxxxxxxxxxxxxxxxxxxxxxxxxxxxxxxx

Instructions:

Step 1: Set the salmon fillets in a pan. Add about ½-inch of water and the lemon juice. Set the pan on the stove over medium heat. Cover and let the fish cook for about 10 minutes.

Step 2: While the salmon is cooking, divide the greens between 2 plates. Lay a slice of cooked salmon on top of the greens.

Step 3: Divide the avocado and strawberries equally between the two plates. Set to the side for the moment.

Step 4: In a small bowl, whisk together the vinegar and oil. Season with salt. This is the dressing.

Step 5: Drizzle the dressing over the salads before serving.

Recipe 14: Cream of Broccoli Soup

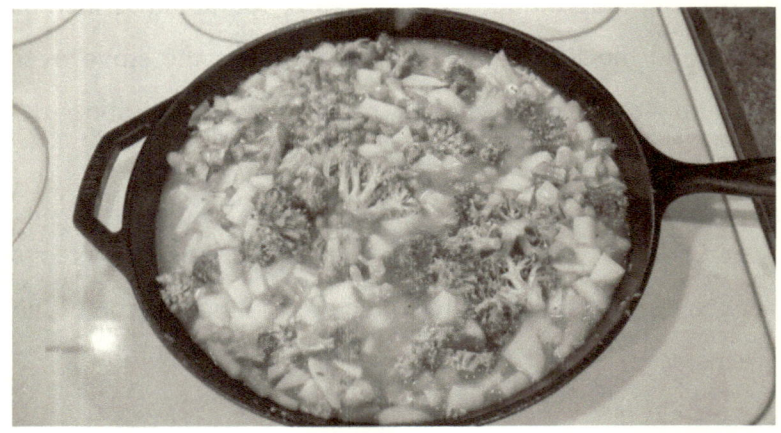

Designed to reduce inflammation and prevent autoimmune disease flare-ups, this cream of broccoli soup is a wonderful meal that will warm you while filling your belly.

Yield: 4

Cooking Time: 35 to 40 minutes

List of Ingredients:

- 2 turnips, peeled and diced
- 1 yellow onion, diced
- 1 head broccoli, diced
- 4 cups chicken stock, low-sodium
- 1 tsp. sea salt
- 2 Tbsp. extra-virgin olive oil

xxxxxxxxxxxxxxxxxxxxxxxxxxxxxxxxxxxxx

Instructions:

Step 1: Add the olive oil to a stockpot. Set the pot on the stove over medium heat. Add the onion and sauté until tender.

Step 2: Stir the chicken stock, turnip, broccoli and salt together in the pot. Cover the pot with a lid and let the mixture come to a boil.

Step 3: Once the mixture is boiling, reduce heat and let simmer for about 20 to 25 minutes.

Step 4: Remove the pot from heat. Using an immersion blender, blend the soup until smooth.

Step 5: Divide the soup between 4 bowls and serve while still warm.

Recipe 15: Mango Shrimp Salad

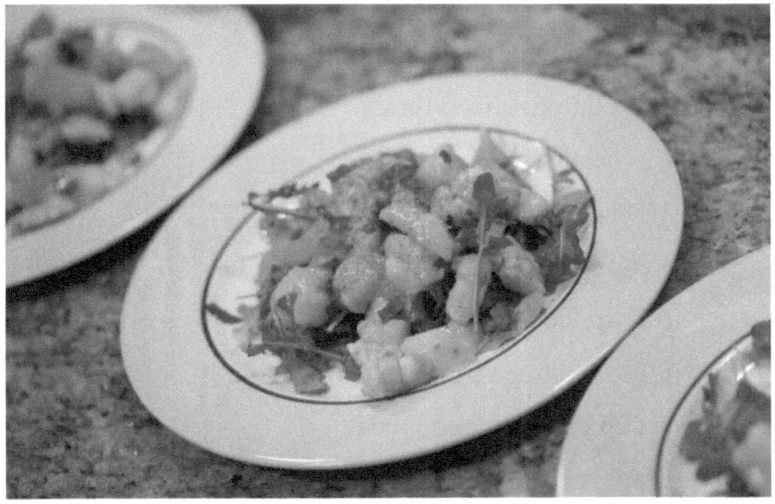

Refreshing with a tropical flavor, this mango and shrimp salad gives you a fun and exciting option for a meal.

Yield: 2

Cooking Time: 15 to 20 minutes

List of Ingredients:

- 1-pound shrimp, deveined, cleaned and tails left on
- 1 cup mango, peeled and diced
- 1 red onion, sliced thinly
- 1 avocado, peeled and diced
- 2 Tbsp. lime juice
- 4 cups mixed greens
- 1 Tbsp. coconut oil
- 1 Tbsp. extra-virgin olive oil
- ½ cup cilantro, chopped
- 1 tsp. salt, kosher or sea

XXXXXXXXXXXXXXXXXXXXXXXXXXXXXXXXXXXXXXXX

Instructions:

Step 1: Add the coconut oil to a skillet and set on the stove over medium heat. Add the shrimp and cook until translucent on all sides of the seafood.

Step 2: While the shrimp is cooking, mix the mango, avocado, onion and cilantro until well combined.

Step 3: In a small bowl, create the dressing by mixing the lime juice, olive oil and salt together. Set to the side for the moment.

Step 4: Divide the mixed greens between serving plates. Add some of the cooked shrimp on top and drizzle with the dressing.

Chapter V - Autoimmune Disease Dinner Recipes

xxxxxxxxxxxxxxxxxxxxxxxxxxxxxxxxxxxxxxxxxx

Recipe 16: Meatloaf

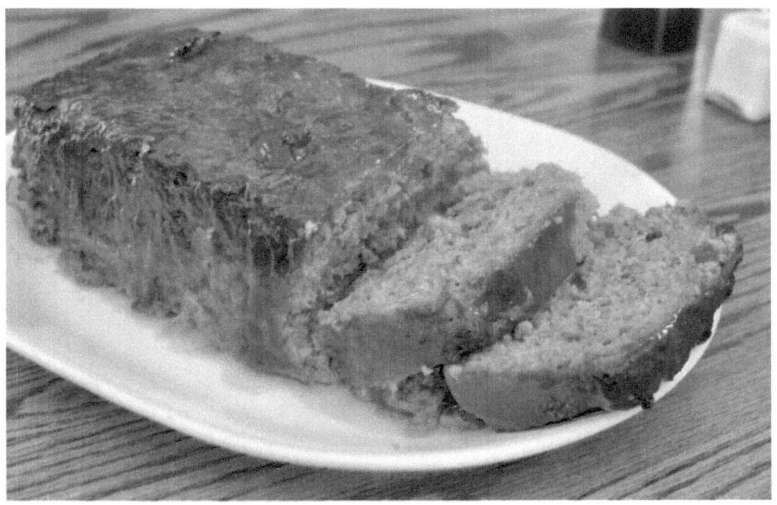

This paleo compliant meatloaf is gluten free yet doesn't skimp on taste. If, however, you have found that red meat increases your inflammation, you may want to skip this recipe.

Yield: 4 to 8

Cooking Time: 60 minutes

List of Ingredients:

- 1 ½ pounds lean ground beef
- 4 ounces tomato sauce
- 1 Tbsp. Worcestershire sauce
- 2 large eggs
- ½ cup pork rinds, crushed
- 1 Tbsp. salt
- 2 ½ Tbsp. chili powder
- 1 Tbsp. garlic pepper seasoning

xxxxxxxxxxxxxxxxxxxxxxxxxxxxxxxxxxxxxxx

Instructions:

Step 1: Turn the oven to 375-degrees and let preheat. Lightly grease the bottom and sides of a loaf pan and set to the side for the moment.

Step 2: In a mixing bowl, knead the beef, pork rinds, tomato sauce, eggs and Worcestershire sauce with your hands.

Step 3: Season the beef mixture with the chili powder, garlic pepper and garlic sauce and knead once again until well incorporated.

Step 4: Press the beef mixture into the prepared loaf pan from Step 1. Place the loaf pan in the preheated oven and bake for about 40 minutes. Remove the pan from the oven and let sit for about 5 minutes.

Step 5: Carefully remove the meatloaf from the pan and set on a serving platter. Slice the meatloaf before serving.

Recipe 17: Italian-Style Pot Roast

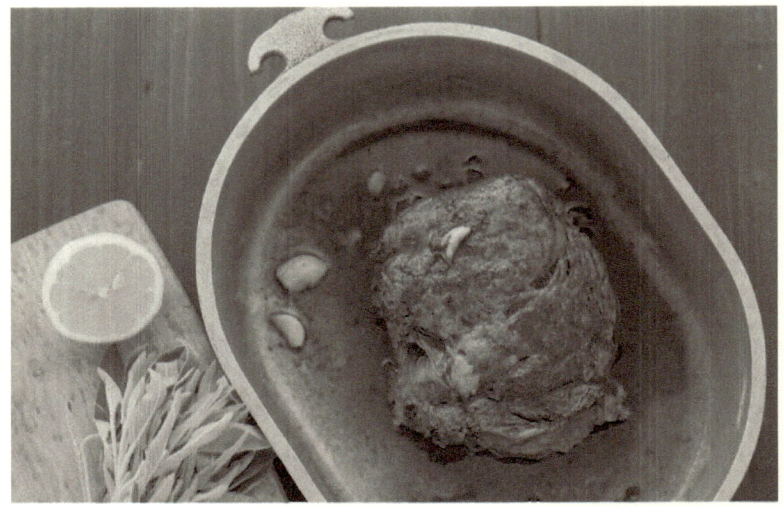

This juicy pot roast is a crowd pleasure and can feed a lot of people with a few tweaks of the ingredients.

Yield: 4

Cooking Time: 5 hours

List of Ingredients:

- 2-pound roast beef, chuck or rump
- 2 Tbsp. + 2 Tbsp. olive oil
- ¾ Tbsp. sea salt
- 2 celery stalks, diced
- 2 carrots, diced
- 1 red onion, diced
- 2 garlic cloves, minced finely
- 1 bay leaf
- 2 Tbsp. sage, minced finely
- ¼ cup parsley, minced finely
- 2 cups red wine vinegar, divided

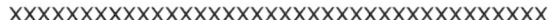

xxxxxxxxxxxxxxxxxxxxxxxxxxxxxxxxxxxxxxxx

Instructions:

Step 1: Trim and discard the fat from the roast before patting the roast dry with some paper towels. Season the roast with sea salt.

Step 2: Heat 2 Tbsp. of olive oil in a stockpot on medium heat. Set the seasoned roast in the pot and sear on all sides. You want the roast to be brown on all sides, which should take about 10 minutes. Remove the seared roast from the pot and set on a platter.

Step 3: Add the remaining 2 Tbsp. of olive oil into the stockpot. Set the pot back on the stove over medium heat. Stir in the celery, onion and carrot and sauté for about 10 minutes. Add the parsley, sage and garlic and stir for another minute or two.

Step 4: Carefully pour 1 ½ cup of the vinegar into the pot and stir. Continue cooking and stirring until the vinegar has almost evaporated completely. Carefully return the seared roast back into the stockpot and coat the roast in the vinegar coated herbs and veggies.

Step 5: Turn the heat under the stockpot up to high. Pour in the remaining vinegar and bay leaf.

Step 6: Let the mixture start to boil before reducing the heat, covering the pot with a lid and letting it simmer for about 3 hours. Make sure to turn and baste the roast every 30 minutes during the simmering process.

Step 7: Turn the heat underneath the pot off and let the mixture rest for about 60 minutes.

Step 8: Remove the roast from the pot and set on a serving platter. Slice the roast and drizzle the juices from the pot overtop the meat before serving.

Recipe 18: Pork Tenderloin

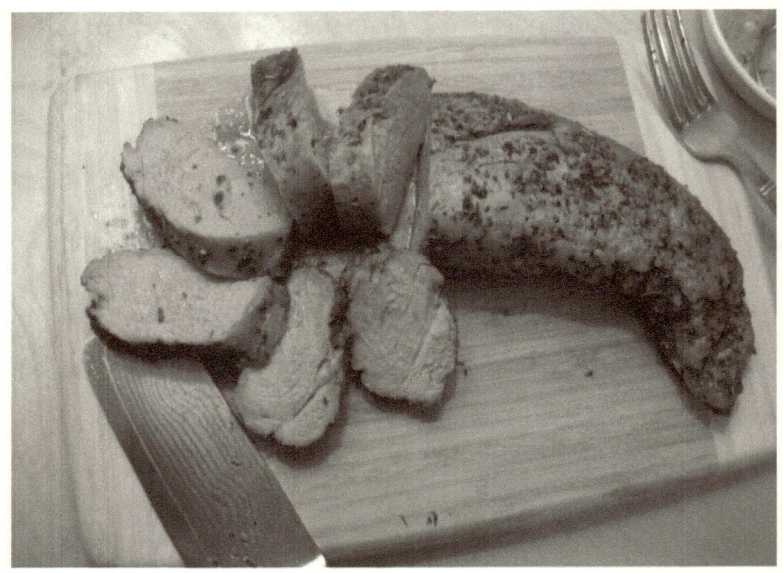

What makes this autoimmune disease diet compliant roasted pork so delicious is the herbs and the homemade apricot sauce.

Yield: 4

Cooking Time: 25 to 30 minutes

List of Ingredients:

- 1 pork tenderloin
- 1 tsp. marjoram
- 1 tsp. rosemary
- 1 tsp. oregano
- 1 tsp. thyme
- 1 tsp. basil
- 1 tsp. sea salt
- ½ tsp. pepper, ground black
- 1 cup apricots, dried
- 1 tsp. apple cider vinegar
- 2/3 cup water

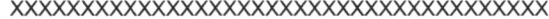

xxxxxxxxxxxxxxxxxxxxxxxxxxxxxxxxxxxxxxxx

Instructions:

Step 1: Turn the oven to 425-degrees and let preheat.

Step 2: Mix the rosemary, oregano, thyme, marjoram, basil, thyme, salt and black pepper together in a small bowl.

Step 3: Rub and press the herb mixture from Step 2 all over and into the pork tenderloin. Lay the seasoned pork on a baking sheet.

Step 4: Place the baking sheet in the preheated oven and let cook for about 15 minutes. Remove the baking sheet from the oven and let the pork rest for about 10 minutes.

Step 5: While the pork is resting, make the apricot sauce by placing the 2/3 cups of water, vinegar and dried apricots in a blender and blend until the mixture is smooth.

Step 6: Pour the sauce from Step 5 into a saucepan and set on the stove over medium heat. Let the sauce cook a bit until it starts to thicken a bit. Make sure to stir constantly to prevent the sauce from burning.

Step 7: Place the cooked pork onto a serving platter and drizzle the apricot sauce over top before serving.

Recipe 19: Sweet & Sour Chicken

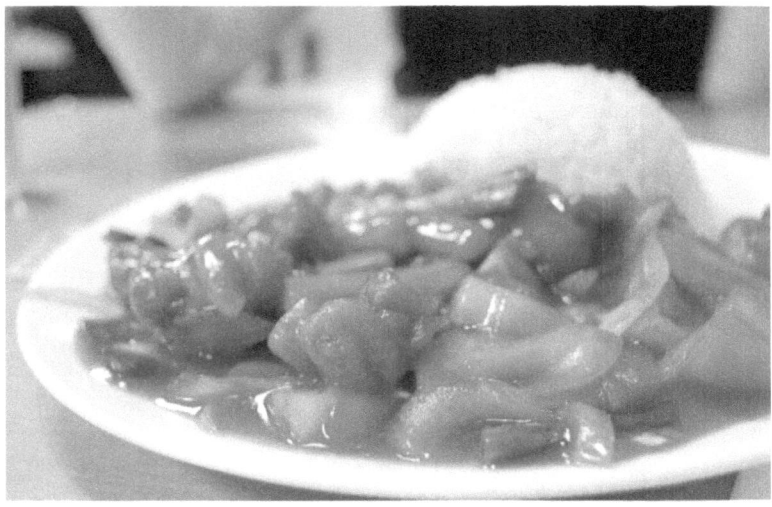

Delicious and compliant with the autoimmune disease diet, this take on the traditional Oriental dish will please everyone in your household!

Yield: 4

Cooking Time: 30 to 35 minutes

List of Ingredients:

- 1-pound chicken breast, skinless and cubed
- 1 cup pineapple, diced
- 1 bunch scallions, diced
- 2 celery stalks, diced
- 2 carrots, diced
- ¼ cup vinegar, apple cider
- ½ pound mushrooms, sliced
- 2 garlic cloves, minced
- 1 inch ginger root, peeled and grated
- 2 Tbsp. coconut oil

xxxxxxxxxxxxxxxxxxxxxxxxxxxxxxxxxxxxxxxxx

Instructions:

Step 1: Place the celery, garlic and onions in a wok and sauté for a few minutes until soft.

Step 2: Add the mushrooms, pineapple, chicken and carrots into the wok and continue to cook for about 6 to 8 minutes.

Step 3: Pour the vinegar into the wok and stir. Cover the wok before turning the heat down to low.

Step 4: Let the mixture cook for about 10 minutes. Remove the wok from heat and let cool for a few minutes before serving.

Recipe 20: Gluten and Grain Free Pizza

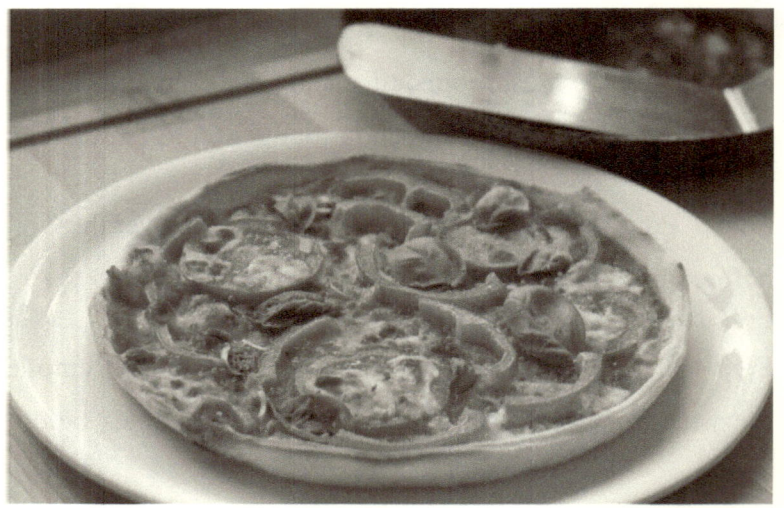

This almond crust chicken pizza is made especially for people following the paleo, anti-inflammatory and autoimmune disease diet.

Yield: 4

Cooking Time: 40 to 45 minutes

Crust Ingredients:

- 4 cups almond flour
- 4 large eggs
- 1 tsp. sea salt
- 4 Tbsp. extra-virgin olive oil

Topping Ingredients:

- 1 can tomato paste
- 2 tomatoes, diced
- 1 bunch basil leaves
- 3 garlic cloves, minced
- 1 chopped onion, yellow or red
- 1-pound chicken breast, cooked and diced

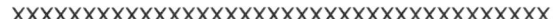

Instructions:

Step 1: Turn the oven to 350-degrees and let preheat.

Step 2: Make the crust by mixing all the crust ingredients together to form the dough. Lay out a piece of parchment paper and lightly grease it with olive oil. Roll the dough out on the paper to the desired thickness. Carefully move the dough and parchment paper onto a pizza tray.

Step 3: Place the pizza tray in the oven and bake for about 12 minutes. Remove from the oven.

Step 4: Spread the tomato paste over the pizza crust. Sprinkle the chopped vegetables and the cubed, cooked chicken over the pizza crust.

Step 5: Place the pizza back in the oven for an additional 12 to 15 minutes.

Step 6: Remove the pizza from the oven and let cook for a few moments before cutting into slices and serving.

Chapter VI - Autoimmune Disease Snack and Dessert Recipes

xxxxxxxxxxxxxxxxxxxxxxxxxxxxxxxxxxxxxxxxxx

Recipe 21: Paleo-Style No Bake Brownie Bits

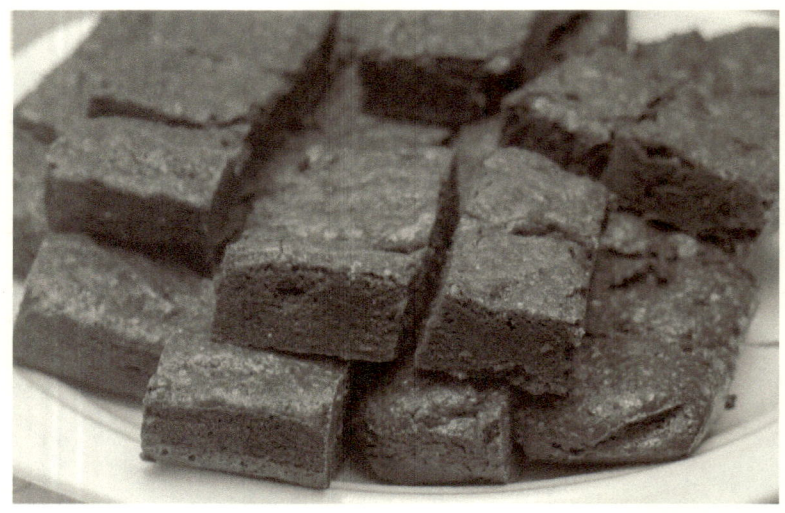

Since these delicious brownie bits are no baked, they can be made in a few minutes. They are also paleo-style so you won't be consuming overly processed ingredients.

Yield: 4 to 5

Cooking Time: 15 minutes

List of Ingredients:

- 1 cup dates, pitted
- 1 ½ cups raw walnuts
- 1/3 cup unsweetened cocoa powder
- 1 tsp. vanilla
- Pinch of salt

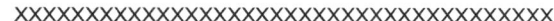

xxxxxxxxxxxxxxxxxxxxxxxxxxxxxxxxxxxxxxxx

Instructions:

Step 1: Prepare a baking sheet by covering it with parchment paper. Set to the side for the moment.

Step 2: Place the raw walnuts into a food processor and pulse until the nuts has a consistency similar to powder.

Step 3: Add the dates, cocoa powder, vanilla and salt to the nut powder and pulse until the mixture is smooth.

Step 4: Using your hands, roll the brownie mixture into small, bite-sized balls. Set the balls on the parchment paper-covered baking sheet. Continue in this manner until you have no more brownie mixture.

Step 5: Consumer the brownie bites or store them in a container in the fridge until ready to eat.

Recipe 22: Cinnamon Apple Crisps

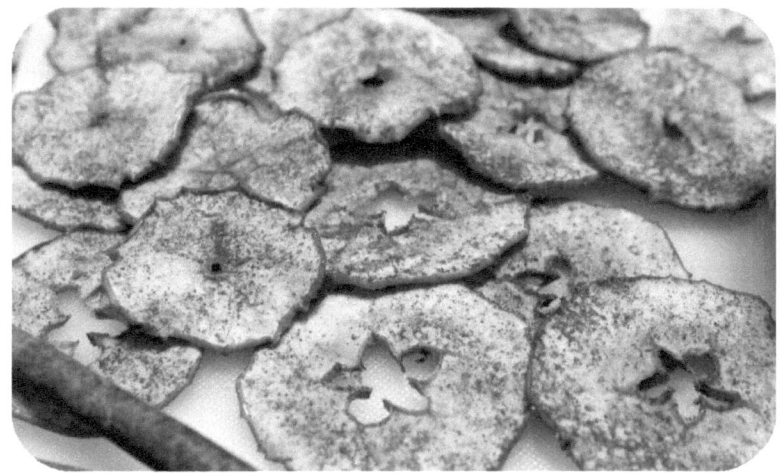

If you're looking for a snack with a bit of sweetness, give these red and green crisps made with two different types of apples and featuring cinnamon.

Yield: 4

Cooking Time: 2 hours 10 minutes

List of Ingredients:

- 2 red apples, such as Gala or McIntosh
- 2 green apples, such as Granny Smith
- ½ tsp. salt, sea or kosher
- 1 tsp. ground cinnamon

XX

Instructions:

Step 1: Turn the oven to 200-degrees and let preheat. Prepare two cookie sheets by lining them with parchment paper. Set to the side for the moment.

Step 2: Core all 4 apples and slice each on into thin rounds.

Step 3: Lay the apple slices in a single layer along the prepared cookie sheets from Step 1.

Step 4: Sprinkle the salt over the apple chips, followed by the ground cinnamon.

Step 5: Bake the seasoned apple chips in the preheated oven for about 60 minutes. Remove the cookie sheets from the oven and flip the apple chips over. Place them back in the oven and bake for an additional 60 minutes.

Step 6: Transfer the apple chips to a rack and let cool. Once cooled, store the apple chips in an airtight container until ready to enjoy.

Recipe 23: Plantain Fries

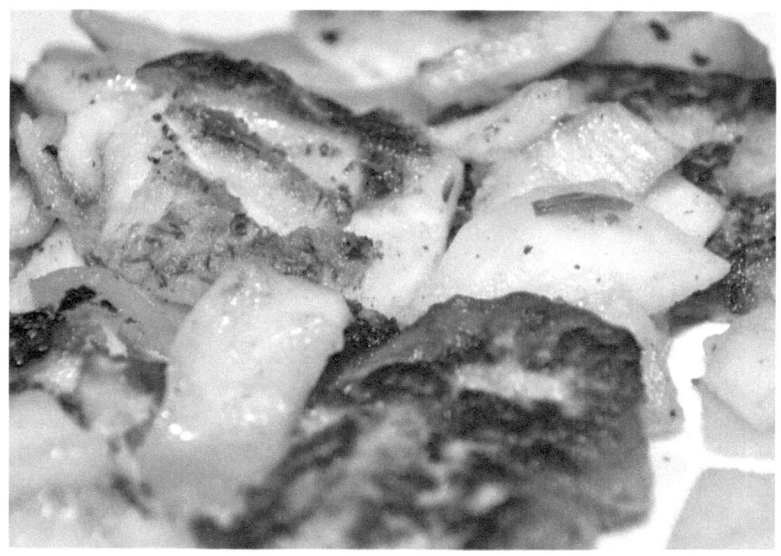

Since potatoes are a common inflammation culprit, you will probably want to eliminate them for your diet and replace them with this delicious and healthier option.

Yield: 1

Cooking Time: 25 to 30 minutes

List of Ingredients:

- 1 green plantain
- ½ lime
- Sea salt, to taste
- Black pepper, to taste
- Coconut oil
- Water

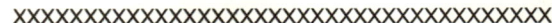

xxxxxxxxxxxxxxxxxxxxxxxxxxxxxxxxxxxxxxx

Instructions:

Step 1: Pour water into a large pot. Add some sea salt and stir. Set the pot on the stove over high heat and bring the water to a boil. Set a saucepan on the stove over medium heat. Add the coconut oil to coat the bottom of the pan.

Step 2: Prepare the plantain by cutting both ends off and cutting down the peel on each side. Remove the peel and discard.

Step 3: Slice the peeled plantain into ¼-inch slices. Carefully place these slices in the boiling water and cook until tender, which should be about 5 minutes.

Step 4: Drain the water from the plantains. Transfer the plantains into the coconut oil coated pan and let cook for about 4 minutes on each one of the fruit's side.

Step 5: Transfer the cooked plantain slices to a paper towel-covered plate and allow the excess coconut oil to drain off.

Step 6: Move the plantain slices onto a serve plate. Season with salt and pepper before drizzling the lime juice over top. Serve while the plantain fries are still warm.

Recipe 24: Coconut and Sea Salt Chips

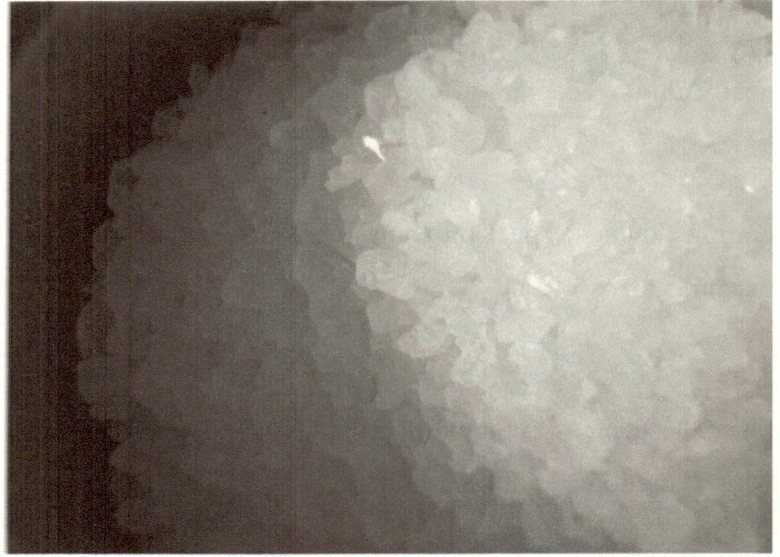

This delicious snack is perfect for at home, as well as a grab and go option. And it only requires 2 ingredients!

Yield: 4 to 6 cups of chips

Cooking Time: 60 minutes

List of Ingredients:

- 1 coconut
- Sea salt

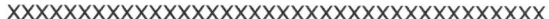

Instructions:

Step 1: Turn the oven to 350-degrees and let preheat. Cover two baking sheets with parchment paper and set to the side for the moment.

Step 2: Grab the coconut and find the softest part of the stem by pressing your thumb into it. Once you have found the softest part, use an ice pick to piece the coconut and let the water drain out.

Step 3: Set the coconut on a baking dish and heat in the oven until the coconut shell starts to crack, which should be about 30 minutes. Set the cooked coconut on a cooling rack and let cool for about 10 minutes.

Step 4: Wrap the cooled coconut in a towel. While holding the coconut, carefully smack it with a hammer until the outer shell starts to crack. The coconut should now have spilt into pieces.

Step 5: Remove the coconut flesh from the shell. If there is darker outer skin left on the coconut, remove it with a vegetable peeler.

Step 6: Rinse the coconut with cool water before patting it dry.

Step 7: Use a vegetable peeler to slice the coconut into varying size strips.

Step 8: Spread the coconut strips along the bottom of the prepared baking sheets from Step 1. Make sure they are spread evenly in a single layer.

Step 9: Place the baking sheets in the oven and bake the coconut strips until they are a lightly toasted, which is 10 or so minutes.

Step 10: Remove the baking sheets from the oven and let the coconut chips cool for several minutes before removing the chips from the baking sheets and transferring them into an airtight container.

Recipe 25: Coconut Ginger Ice Cream

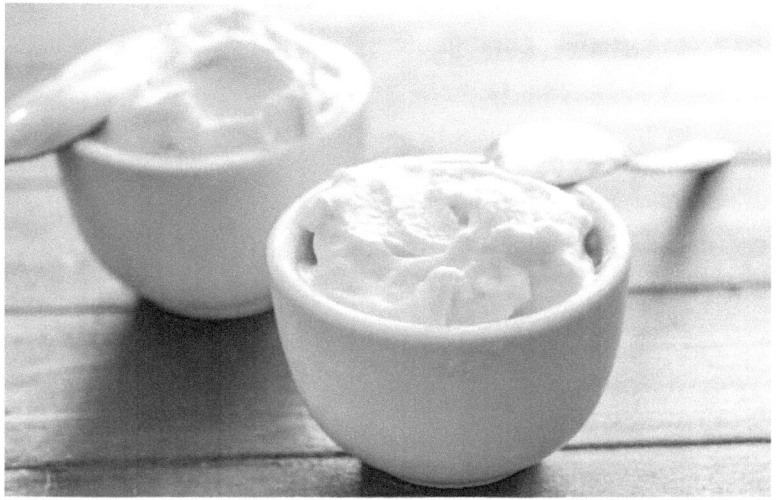

Dairy is a cause of inflammation for a lot of people. If you are one of them, you can still enjoy ice cream by making your own using coconut milk instead of traditional dairy.

Yield: 4 to 6

Cooking Time: 25 minutes

List of Ingredients:

- 2 tins coconut milk
- 120 grams dates, pitted
- 15 grams grated ginger
- 3 Tbsp. vanilla
- 3 Tbsp. gelatin
- Sea salt, pinch

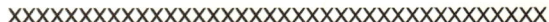

XXXXXXXXXXXXXXXXXXXXXXXXXXXXXXXXXXXXXXX

Instructions:

Step 1: Prepare the dates by steaming them over boiling water. You want to remove as much of the moisture from the fruits as possible. Remove the steamed dates and set to the side for the moment.

Step 2: Place the coconut milk, vanilla, ginger, gelatin, pinch of sea salt and the steamed dates from Step 1 into a blender. Blend the mixture until smooth.

Step 3: Transfer the mixture from the blender to a container with a lid. Place the container in the fridge for 35 minutes.

Step 4: Transfer the chilled mixture into your ice cream maker. Make the ice cream according to the instructions for your brand of ice cream maker.

Step 5: Consumer the ice cream immediately or place in the freezer for several minutes to firm it up a bit.

About the Author

Heston Brown is an accomplished chef and successful e-book author from Palo Alto California. After studying cooking at The New England Culinary Institute, Heston stopped briefly in Chicago where he was offered head chef at some of the city's most prestigious restaurants. Brown decide that he missed the rolling hills and sunny weather of California and moved back to his home state to open up his own catering company and give private cooking classes.

Heston lives in California with his beautiful wife of 18 years and his two daughters who also have aspirations to follow in their father's footsteps and pursue careers in the culinary arts. Brown is well known for his delicious fish and chicken dishes and teaches these recipes as well as many others to his students.

When Heston gave up his successful chef position in Chicago and moved back to California, a friend suggested he use the internet to share his recipes with the world and so he did! To date, Heston Brown has written over 1000 e-books that contain recipes, cooking tips, business strategies for catering companies and a self-help book he wrote from personal experience.

He claims his wife has been his inspiration throughout many of his endeavours and continues to be his partner in business as well as life. His greatest joy is having all three women in his life in the kitchen with him cooking their favourite meal while his favourite jazz music plays in the background.

Author's Afterthoughts

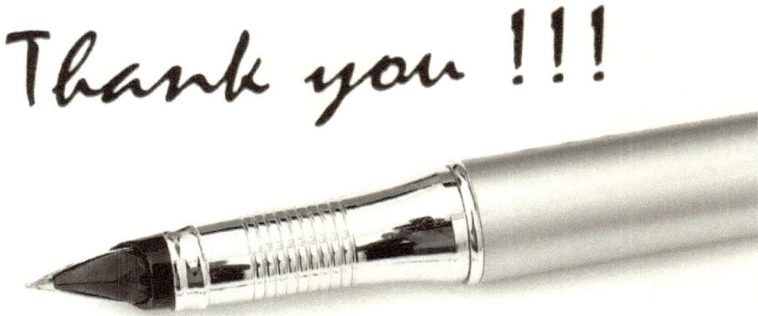

Thank you to all the readers who invested time and money into my book! I cherish every one of you and hope you took the same pleasure in reading it as I did in writing it.

Out of all of the books out there, you chose mine and for that I am truly grateful. It makes the effort worth it when I know my readers are enjoying my work from beginning to end.

Please take a few minutes to write an Amazon review so that others can benefit from your opinions and insight. Your review will help countless other readers make an informed choice

Thank you so much,

Heston Brown

www.ingramcontent.com/pod-product-compliance
Lightning Source LLC
Chambersburg PA
CBHW02 228280526
45784CB00005B/2016